Basics of Nutrition

The First Book You Need To Read To Begin A Healthy Lifestyle

Introduction

I want to thank you and congratulate you for downloading the book, *"Basics of Nutrition: The First book You need to read to begin a healthy lifestyle"*.

This book contains proven steps and strategies on how to maintain a perfect health and live a healthy lifestyle with less stress.

This book contains about six chapters all directed towards living a healthy lifestyle. All you need to know about nutrition, the right food to eat on a daily basics and so much more that would be very helpful for you.

Thanks again for downloading this book, I hope you enjoy it!

Chapter 1

What is Nutrition?

Before embarking on this journey to a healthy lifestyle, there are some things one must know. The few things forms the basics. You have to know what nutrition is, what health is as well as the connection between the health and nutrition.

Nutrition is simple terms, involves what we take into our body that is what we eat. It has to do with food. We all know the kind of food we eat, very dependent on the location we are. An American's food would definitely be different from that of an Iranian. The end goal of taking in food into the body is for nourishment.

Nutrition according to science is the science that interprets the interaction of nutrients and other substances in food in relation to maintenance, **growth**, **reproduction**, **health** and disease of an organism. It includes **food intake**, **absorption**, **assimilation**, **biosynthesis**, **catabolism**, and **excretion**.

Nutrition involves so many processes as mentioned above as well as it has direct link with some of them such Growth, reproduction and so on (check the words written above in bold letters). Let's take a look at these words.

Growth simply means increase in size, weight and height. It is the act of getting bigger or taller. Nutrition, however contributes to one's growth. Proper and good Nutrition would enhance adequate growth while poor nutrition would definitely lead to poor growth. We would talk more on this later in this book.

Reproduction is the process of procreation. It is a biological process that involves the production of new individuals 'offspring' by the parents- mother and father. In simple terms, it involves a sexual relationship between a male and a female leading to production of young ones. Without the proper growth and development of the necessary reproductive organs, reproduction would definitely not be possible. This solely depends on Nutrition.

Finally, health is also a word that is directly linked to nutrition. Health according WHO (World Health Organization) is a state of physical, mental and social well-being and not just the absence of diseases or infirmities. This simply means that you're not healthy only when you're not sick. Healthiness encompasses three aspects- the physical, the mental as well as the social. Proper and adequate Nutrition equals good health.

The Processes Involved in Nutrition

As listed above, nutrition involves a few processes which includes:

- Food intake
- Absorption and Assimilation
- Biosynthesis
- Catabolism and
- Excretion

When we talk about food intake, we simply mean eating or consumption of food. This is first step in the process of nutrition. It involves passing food through the mouth into the body. It may involve chewing and/or swallowing depending on the kind of food you are taking in. We all know this, since no one was really taught how to eat or where to put the food. We just learnt how to do these things by default. After the intake of food through the mouth, the food then goes directly into the body.

Before moving on to absorption, let's talk about classes of food. Food can be classified into about six (6) main classes. It includes Carbohydrates, Protein, fats, vitamins, minerals and water.

Carbohydrates

This is a class of food that basically provides us with energy when taken. Examples include rice, bread, potatoes and so on.

Protein

Proteins on the hand, is a class of food that helps in body building, repair of worn-out tissues as well as building of new tissues, hormones, enzymes and antibodies. Examples include meat, milk, fish, eggs and so on.

Fats

This class of food is type that provides the body with enough insulation, more energy as well as protection. Examples include margarine, butter, cheese and so on.

Vitamins

This kind of food helps in the facilitation of other nutrients. It also assists in the regulation of growth and production of hormones. Examples include vegetables and fruits.

Minerals

This kind assists in the building of bones and teeth, proper functioning of the muscles as well as contributes to nervous system activity. Examples include meat, milk, banana, seafood, eggs and so on.

Water

Everyone should be familiar with this class of food, although most people might not know that it is part of the classes of food. Water is important aspect of food and it should never be ignored. Water helps in the dissolution of food substances as well as in the conveyance of nutrients in the body. Sometimes when you eat, you notice that the even though you took a drink or juice with the food, you still feel thirsty for water. That is how important water is. Water also aids digestion of food, regulation of body temperature (homeostasis) and removal of waste materials.

Getting to know how your body absorbs the food taken into the body would help on this journey to living a healthy lifestyle. Absorption simply involves the process whereby food digested is absorbed by the blood and distributed in the proportion to the other areas or parts of the body. The first step in absorption of food is digestion. Food has to be digested first before being absorbed into the blood. It takes place through osmosis or diffusion.

The human body absorbs two kinds of nutrients: The Macronutrients and Micronutrients.

Macronutrients are the kind of foods taking into the body that provides us with energy directly such as Carbohydrates, fats and protein. They are referred to as 'Macro' nutrients because they are required in the body in large quantities.

Micronutrients on the other hand are those kind of nutrients that help in the provision of energy but not indirectly. They serve as <u>catalyst</u>.

They are referred to as 'micro' nutrients because they are required in the body in small quantities. Examples include vitamins and minerals.

We can't talk of nutrition and not mention excretion. Excretion is simply the removal of metabolic waste from the body. After digestion, it is not all the food taking into the body would be utilized by the body.

In this chapter, we have successfully discussed on the basic things we need to know about Nutrition like the classes of food we have, what nutrition is and so on.

Chapter 2

Importance of One's Health

Health this refers to a state of complete physical, mental and social well being, it is not just the absence of disease and infirmity. Health may also be defined as the ability to adapt and manage physical, mental and social challenges through out life.

Factor of good health include the physical social and economic environment, genetics, relationships, education and lifestyle. Good health is central to handling stress and living a long active and productive life. It's not a coincidence that The 3rd sustainable development goal is Good health and well-being. The goal is to ensure healthy lives for all at all ages as it important to building prosperous societies.

Access to good health and well being is a human right. Health care exist to assist in the maintenance of this optimal state of wellness. Good health of mind and body and access to standard health care facilities for all is of great importance that's why the sustainable development goal hopes to achieve this task by making health care available and affordable to everyone and not just the wealthy.

Being healthy means that your body and mind are working as they are supposed to. Being healthy can not be over emphasized, it means finding out what works best for you and your lifestyle, making informed choices that can help energize you, treat your body with care and fuel yourself with the right nutrients. Being healthy means looking good, feeling fit, being confident, strong, active and productive.

A healthy diet, exercise, proper care of the body and environment, screening for diseases and coping strategies can help a person maintain a healthy.

In playing our various roles in the society it is important that we are healthy, individually its our responsibility to keep a healthy lifestyle, taking good care of our body, mind, emotions and environment as our personal hygiene is important, our social environment and public cleanliness is also important for individual health.

Good health is important and beneficial especially for someone who wants to be productive and effective in the society. A clear distinction is often made between 'mind' and 'body'. But when considering mental health and physical health, the two should not be thought of as separate.

Poor physical health can lead to an increased risk of developing mental health problems. Similarly, poor mental health can negatively impact on physical health, leading to an increased risk of some conditions.

The associations between mental and physical health are: Poor mental health is a risk factor for chronic physical conditions; People with serious mental health conditions are at high risk of experiencing chronic physical conditions; People with chronic physical conditions are at risk of developing poor mental health.

Physical Health this means your body is functioning as it is supposed to, without pain or discomfort or lack of capabilities. Physical health is of Prime importance, being physically ill can be an impediment to one's productive life. Injuries, stress, loss of appetite, general weakness of the body are prominent symptoms for most sickness and diseases would prevent one from being able to work, move or eat. If you feel physically fit and healthy, it would be easy to lead a normal and productive lifestyle.

Being physically healthy starts with good nutrition and proper exercise of the muscles and joints to prevent conditions like osteoporosis as it has effect on developing proper muscles and bones. Physical activities or exercise can improve your health and reduce the risk of developing several diseases like cardiovascular diseases, diabetes, manage your weight better and makes you feel relaxed with more energy and a better mood

Mental Health refers to emotional health. Mental health is a level of psychological well-being or the absence of mental illness. Mental health includes our ability to enjoy life, our emotional, psychological, and social well-being. It affects how we think, feel, and act. It also helps determine how we handle stress, relate to others, and make choices. Mental health is important at every stage of life, from childhood and adolescence through adulthood.

Many factors contribute to mental health problems, including: Biological factors, such as genes or brain chemistry; Life experiences such as trauma or abuse; Family history of mental health problems.

Positive mental health allows people to: Be sociable, connecting with others; Stay positive; Get physically active; Helping others; Getting enough sleep; Realize their full potential; Cope with the stresses of life; Work productively; Make meaningful contributions to their communities.

Some of the most common and frequently reported mental illnesses include depression and bipolar disorders, Anxiety, Stress, Memory Loss, Alzheimer's Disease, Mood Disorders, including seasonal affective disorder, schizophrenia, dementia, and eating disorders.

Depression is the number one cause of disability worldwide and is one of the most significant contributors to the global burden of disease, greatly impacting individuals and their families mentally, physically, socially, and financially. Mental illness affects everyone no matter their race, gender, culture, age, ethnicity, or sexual orientation.

Maintaining mental health is not as specific as maintaining physical health. Building positive energy is a way of forming the right mental attitude, Staying positive is not easy but being negative is counter productive as it gives no solution to the problem at hand and wastes your time and energy worrying and complaining about everything that's not right. Keeping away from toxic substances, relationships and environment is necessary to maintain a healthy lifestyle. Toxic situations can be avoided by simply leaving the scene, apologizing, or keeping such relationship at arms length. Toxic situations have detrimental effects to the body and mind, abuse are not only physical but can also be mental.

Toxic substances and prohibited drugs like cocaine, heroine, should be avoided. Self medication is not advised, alcohol intake should be reduced. These substances are harmful to the body and mind and even though the result are necessarily not immediate it could have detrimental effects on the person in the not so long future.

Taking care of ourselves and environment would reduce the amount of time and resource spent in treating a particular problem if we can prevent its occurrence.

You should learn to deal with problems through informed health care practices. Visit a doctor or a hospital.

Chapter 3

Essential Nutrients For the Body

In chapter one, we have took a little time to lay a foundation of the basics of nutrition: what nutrition really is, types of nutrients that is Macro and Micronutrients and so on. We also said a little about the main classes of the food we have. Well, in this chapter we want to dive into the essential nutrients that our body needs for daily maintenance of perfect health.

What are Essential Nutrients?

Essential nutrients simply means what our body needs on a daily in order to maintain good health. Do not forget that health encompasses three aspects- physical, mental and social and any aspect left out would mean the opposite.

We have mentioned some of these nutrients in chapter one and we just going to elaborate more on them. Let's dive in!

There is a difference between 'just eating' and 'eating right'. Most people just eat whatever they want to eat. They probably have no idea on the fact that there are nutrients that we shouldn't do without on a daily basics. These nutrients are tagged essential nutrients needed in the body. They include:

Carbohydrates

Most people try to avoid this category of food because it has been termed the kind of food that makes one fat and heavy. Most especially, the ladies that would like to keep in shape and not fat. Carbohydrate is an essential nutrient needed by the body in large quantities (Macronutrients). It is broken down into glucose which then provides energy for the brain and the other parts of the body.

Carbohydrate is present in a lot of healthy foods we have today. An example is fruits. It also helps in the maintenance and regulation of sugar level in the blood. We have Simple carbohydrates as well as complex carbohydrates. Simple carbohydrates as the name implies when taken in breaks down easily within a few hours while complex carbohydrates takes a while to break down.

We should know that carbohydrates are important nutrients in the body that should not ignored or abstained from all in the name of keeping in shape. It contributes to the proper functioning of the brain and other parts of the body.

According to health practitioners and nutritionists, there are sources of carbohydrates that are healthier than the other. It is advisable to eat carbs such as whole grains, fresh fruits and vegetables instead of refined and industrialized products. It has also being established that carbohydrates should make up of up to 60% of one's daily intake.

Failure to consume the proper and adequate proportion of carbohydrates daily can lead to what we call 'hypoglycemia'. Hypoglycemia is also know has low blood sugar. It occurs when the level of glucose in the blood reduces beyond normal. It can lead to tiredness, fainting, weakness and hunger.

Eating less than 120 calories in a day can lead to a condition called Ketosis. This occurs as a result accumulation of ketones- partially broken down fats. This could lead to serious health problems such as nausea, bad breath, mental fatigue, kidney stones as well as pains and swellings in the joints. You can actually eat carbohydrates and not get fat by eating sources of carbohydrates that are low in calories such as vegetables and so on.

Proteins

This is a very essential nutrient that should be included in our every day meal. It has a critical implication in our body if not taken adequately. Protein is responsible for the repair of worn-out tissues as well as the production or manufacturing of new body tissues and other important constituents needed in the body- hormones, antibodies and others. It also assists in the building of the body.

These proteins when taken in are broken down into small units known as amino acids. We have about 20 amino acids required by the body in which 9 of them- Histidine, Isoleucine, Leucine, Lysine, Methionine, Phenylalanine, Threonine, Tryptophan and Valine cannot be produced in the body. They can only be gotten by consuming the sources of proteins we have such as dairy, nuts, meats and so on.

Protein should be included in your everyday diet (30%) as it is a crucial nutrient required in the body.

Fats

Like carbohydrates, this type of nutrients avoided most people, especially the ladies and 'slay Queen'. Even its name alone is enough to scare them away real fast. However, fat is also an essential and crucial nutrient required by the human body on a daily. It helps in the provision of energy like carbohydrates. It has been established by some medical and health practitioners that fats provide more energy than carbohydrates.

Fats also contribute to the human body by helping in blood clotting, absorption of vitamins and minerals, movement of muscle, and many other functions. Too much of fat consumption can put at risk such as development of heart and kidney diseases. According to WHO, only 30% of healthy fat should be included daily meal. Yes, we have unhealthy fats- those present in processed and baked food. These kind of fats should not be consumed but avoided strictly as they can increase the risk of health problems.

Consumption of healthy fats has a lot of benefits some of which include: Decrease in the risk of Diabetes and arthritis, enhances brain function and so on. Examples of Healthy fats include: vegetable oil, nuts, seeds and so on

Vitamins

Vitamins is also an essential Micronutrients required by the human body. We have about 13 types of vitamins, all with one function or

Vitamins

Vitamin Name	Major Functions	Deficiency Effects	Toxicity Effects	Food Sources
A Retinol, retinal, Retinoic acid, (Beta carotene)	Vision, immunity, reproduction and growth	Blindness, infections, stunted growth	Bone fractures, liver damage, birth defects	Fortified milk, eggs, liver (dark green leafy and yellow/orange vegetables)
D Cholecalciferol	Bone growth and maintenance, absorption of calcium	Rickets, osteomalacia	Calcium imbalance	Sunlight, fortified milk, fatty fish, eggs, liver
E Tocopherol	Antioxidant, protects cell membranes	Red blood cell breakage, nerve damage	Interferes with blood-clotting drugs	Vegetable and seed/nut oils, seeds and nuts, wheat germ and whole grains
K Phylloquinone	Blood clotting, bone health	Hemorrhage	None reported	Dark leafy greens, cabbage family, liver
B1 Thiamin	Energy metabolism	Beriberi, neurological problems	None reported	Whole and enriched grain products, leafy greens, pork
B2 Riboflavin	Energy metabolism	Inflammation of the mouth, skin	None reported	Whole and enriched grain products, milk products
B3 Niacin	Energy metabolism	Pellagra	Niacin flush, liver damage, impaired glucose tolerance	Whole and enriched grain products, protein-rich foods
B5 Pantothenic acid	Protein, fat and carbohydrate metabolism	Extremely rare	Mild intestinal distress	Almost all foods, especially avocadoes, broccoli, meats
B6 Pyridoxine, pyridoxal, pyridoxamine	Protein and fat metabolism	Scaly dermatitis, anemia, convulsions	Nerve degeneration	Protein-rich foods
B7 Biotin	Protein, fat and carbohydrate metabolism; beneficial to hair, skin and nails	Extremely rare	Unlikely	Egg yolk, liver, peanuts; also produced by gut bacteria
B9 Folate, folic acid, folacin	Helps make DNA for new cells, activates B12	Anemia, birth defects	Masks a B12 deficiency	Fortified grain products, vegetables, legumes
B12 Cobalamin	Helps make DNA for new cells, activates folate, protects nerve cells	Anemia, irreversible nerve damage and paralysis	None reported	Meat, fish, poultry, eggs, milk products
C Ascorbic acid	Antioxidant, collagen synthesis, immune function	Scurvy	Diarrhea	Fruits and vegetables

the other which must not be neglected. If neglected, there are consequences involved. The vitamins we have includes:

The table above shows the types of vitamins, their major functions in the human body, its deficiency when not taken in the right proportion as well as its food sources. Take a lots of fruits, as much as possible per day as they contain great amount of vitamins.

Although, it required in small quantities in the body but that doesn't make it less important or essential.

Minerals

Like vitamins, minerals are also very important micronutrients required in small amount by the body. You should know that failure take these nutrients would attracts some consequences. We have

ESSENTIAL MINERALS

MINERALS	SOURCES	FUNCTIONS	DEFICIENCY	DAILY REQUIREMENT
IRON HAEM NON HAEM	Liver, meat, poultry, fish Cereals, leafy veg, jaggery	Hb formation, brain dev, temperature regulation	Anaemia, impaired cell-mediated immunity	Males=0.84mg Woman=2.8mg Preg.=3.5mg Lactation:2.4mg
CALCIUM	Milk & milk products, eggs, fish, leafy veg, cereals, millets	Bones & teeth, blood coagulation, muscle contraction	Rickets, osteomalacia	600 mg/day
PHOSPHOR US	vegetables	Bones & teeth, Other metabolisms	rare	Equal to calcium
FLOURINE	Drinking water, Sea fish, cheese, tea	Mineralisation of bones, Dental enamel	Dental caries	0.5 to 0.8 mg per litre of water
IODINE	Sea foods, Cod liver oil, milk, vegetables, cereals	Thyroid hormone synthesis	Hypothyroidism, Retarded physical & mental dev	150 mcg / day Preg: 250 mcg/day

different kinds of minerals with their various functions in the body. Some of these minerals include:

The table above shows the essential minerals required by the body, its functions, deficiencies as well as required daily intake.

In this chapter, we have successfully established and discussed the essential nutrients our body requires in order to maintain good health at all times such as Carbohydrates, proteins, fats, minerals and vitamins. We also mentioned that the amount that should be taken in per day. This is because some of these nutrients, if taken in too much might lead to problem because they are required in small quantities.

Chapter 4

Balanced diet

In this book so far, we have been able to successfully treat some core aspects that we need to pay attention to while trying to live a healthy lifestyle. While trying to maintain an healthy lifestyle, you need to mostly consider what you're eating.

Apart from what you take into your body system, there are some other things that can contribute to your health both positively and negatively. For example, your state of mind can determine whether you are healthy or not. Don't forget the definition of health according WHO which says, ***'health is state of physical, mental and social well-being and not just the absence of diseases'***. If you're depressed and cannot sleep, you're not healthy. It is not only food that makes you healthy. Sometimes, of you're sad or let's say poor, you might be able to eat. If you can't eat, growth might be delayed and so on.

It is true that we have essential nutrients that our body requires, some in large quantities (Macronutrients) and some in small quantities (Micronutrients), however these foods should be taken in proportions daily in order to ensure daily maintenance of one's health. This is where balanced diet comes in.

This chapter emphasizes on what we call balanced diet, it basically teaches us the proportion of each food nutrient that should be included in one's diet on a daily basics. We would take a lot at its importance as well as how to achieve it. Let dive into the details.

What is balanced diet?

Diet can be referred to as anything taken in or consumed habitually. Balanced diet simply refers to a diet involving all the essential nutrients in the right proportion. Essential Nutrients including carbohydrates, protein, minerals, vitamins, fats, all included in the right proportions. Since there is balance diet, we can also have unbalanced diet that is when the diet does not include all the essential nutrients in the right proportion.

Note that all the essential nutrients are very important such that when one nutrient is lacking in our diet (body) there might be consequences which might lead to unhealthiness in a way or the other.

In order to maintain a healthy lifestyle nutritionally, you need to include water in your diet. Water is a very essential constituent that shouldn't not be missing. First thing in the morning, when you wake, water should be the first thing you should drink. Water makes you hydrated at all times, makes your skin fresh. It also aids digestion as well as easy distribution of nutrients in the body system. According to nutritionist and professionals in the field of nutrition, it is advisable to take about 64 ounces of water per day for both men and women.

Balanced Diet for Men and Women

For a moderately active individual who works between 8-12 hours per day, in order to keep or maintain a healthy lifestyle, health experts (nutritionist) have advised that men should take as much as 2500 calories and women 2000 calories per day. The number of calories per day can be reduced for less active individuals. A number of works involves a lot of energy in order to carry out their work effectively such as construction workers, wrestlers, athletes and so on. In order to maintain perfect health, protein should be included into your daily diet. For men, 55g per day while for women 50g per day; carbohydrates should not be more than 300g per day for men and about 250g for women; fats also should not be more than 90-95g per day. Too much of fats can lead to severe heart or kidney problem as mentioned earlier. Other nutrients or constituents should also be in check such as sugar (120g per day) and salt (6g per day). Breakfast is a very important meal of the day, you can make your breakfast a protein meal which would sustain till lunch, not too heavy but sustainable such as Scrambled Omelette toast topper, one-pan summer eggs and so on. At lunch you can eat a little mix between protein and carbohydrates to ensure energy as well maintenance of blood sugar. For example you can eat burger, sandwich contain lean meat, salmon or turkey, bread and so on. Dinner should be a heavy meal, carbs free but rich in fiber and vitamins such a vegetable or salad meal and so on.

Chapter 5

Healthy Eating

Healthy eating is not a phrase that refers to strict dietary limitations, or the need to lose weight in order to be unrealistically thin, or depriving yourself of the foods you love or junk food just because you think that's what's making you add weight.

Rather, it's about feeling great, having more energy, improving your health, and boosting your mood. If you feel overwhelmed by all the conflicting nutrition and diet advice out there, you're not alone. It seems that for every expert who tells you a certain food is good for you, you'll find another saying exactly the opposite. But by using these simple tips, you can cut through the confusion and learn how to create—and stick to—a tasty, varied, and nutritious diet that is as good for your mind as it is for your body.

What is a healthy diet?

A healthy diet is a diet that helps to maintain or improve overall health. A healthy diet provides the body with essential nutrition: fluid, macronutrients, micronutrients, and adequate calories.

Eating a healthy diet doesn't have to be overly complicated. While some specific foods or nutrients have been shown to have a beneficial effect on mood, it's your overall dietary pattern that is most important. The cornerstone of a healthy diet pattern should be to replace processed food with real food whenever possible. Eating food that is as close as possible to the way nature made it can make a huge difference to the way you think, look, and feel.

For people who are healthy, a healthy diet is not complicated and contains mostly fruits, vegetables, and whole grains, and includes little to no processed food and sweetened beverages. The requirements for a healthy diet can be met from a variety of plant-based and animal-based foods, although a non-animal source of vitamin B12 is needed for those following a vegan diet.

Various nutrition guides are published by medical and governmental institutions to educate individuals on what they should be eating to be healthy. Nutrition facts labels are also mandatory in some countries to allow consumers to choose between foods based on the components relevant to health. A healthy lifestyle includes getting exercise every day along with eating a healthy diet. A healthy lifestyle may lower disease risks, such as obesity, heart disease, type 2 diabetes, hypertension and cancer.

There are specialized healthy diets, called medical nutrition therapy, for people with various diseases or conditions. There are also prescientific ideas about such specialized diets, as in dietary therapy in traditional Chinese medicine.

Medical nutrition therapy (MNT) is a therapeutic approach to treating medical conditions and their associated symptoms via the use of a specifically tailored diet devised and monitored by a medical doctor physician or registered dietitian nutritionist (RDN). The diet is based upon the patient's medical record, physical examination, functional examination and dietary history.[citation needed]

The role of MNT when administered by a physician or dietitian nutritionist (RDN) is to reduce the risk of developing complications in pre-existing conditions such as type 2 diabetes as well as ameliorate the effects any existing conditions such as high cholesterol. Many medical conditions either develop or are made worse by an improper or unhealthy diet. Studies have shown that people who eat diets rich in fruits, vegetables, nuts, whole grains, and fish consume higher levels of vitamins and minerals from these foods and also have a lower risk of many diseases, including heart disease, stroke, diabetes, and cancers. On the other hand, trials testing the effect of selected vitamins or minerals as pill supplements have mostly shown very little influence on health. The main exception may be fish oil supplements, for which some trials show a lower risk of heart disease and possibly vitamin D.

Does your diet deliver sufficient amounts of vitamins and minerals? Eat real food. That's the essence of today's nutrition message. Our knowledge of nutrition has come full circle, back to eating food that is as close as possible to the way nature made it. The foods you eat have the power to help you live a longer, healthier life. Choose the right foods and you'll fuel your body with the nutrients it needs to prevent nearly every disease and dysfunction from cataracts, infertility, and neurodegenerative conditions to cardiovascular disease and cancer.

Just as the right foods can help your health, the wrong foods can increase your risk of heart disease, type 2 diabetes, high blood pressure, and more.

The Building Blocks to Healthy Eating

The secret to nature is balance, so also is the secret to healthy eating. We all need a balance of all the basic nutrients in our diet including protein, fat, carbohydrates, fiber, vitamins, and minerals. These nutrients help to sustain a healthy body. You don't need to eliminate certain categories of food from your diet, but rather select the healthiest options from each category.

Protein gives you the energy to get up and go—and keep going—while also supporting mood and cognitive function. Too much protein can be harmful to people with kidney disease, but the latest research suggests that many of us need more high-quality protein, especially as we age. That doesn't mean you have to eat more animal products—a variety of plant-based sources of protein each day can ensure your body gets all the essential protein it needs.

Fat. Not all fats are the same. While bad fats can wreck your diet and increase your risk of certain diseases, good fats protect your brain and heart. In fact, healthy fats—such as omega-3s—are vital to your physical and emotional health. Including more healthy fat in your diet can help improve your mood, boost your well-being, and even trim your waistline.

Fiber. Eating foods high in dietary fiber (grains, fruit, vegetables, nuts, and beans) can help you stay regular and lower your risk for heart disease, stroke, and diabetes. It can also improve your skin and even help you to lose weight

Calcium. As well as leading to osteoporosis, not getting enough calcium in your diet can also contribute to anxiety, depression, and sleep difficulties. Whatever your age or gender, it's vital to include calcium-rich foods in your diet, limit those that deplete calcium, and get enough magnesium and vitamins D and K to help calcium do its job.

Carbohydrates are one of your body's main sources of energy. But most should come from complex, unrefined carbs (vegetables, whole grains, fruit) rather than sugars and refined carbs. Cutting back on white bread, pastries, starches, and sugar can prevent rapid spikes in blood sugar, fluctuations in mood and energy, and a build-up of fat, especially around your waistline.

Chapter 6

Tips to Healthy Eating

Switching to a healthy diet doesn't have to be an all or nothing proposition. You don't have to be perfect, you don't have to completely eliminate foods you enjoy, and you don't have to change everything all at once—that usually only leads to cheating or giving up on your new eating plan.

A better approach is to make a few small changes at a time. Keeping your goals modest can help you achieve more in the long term without feeling deprived or overwhelmed by a major diet overhaul. Think of planning a healthy diet as a number of small, manageable steps—like adding a salad to your diet once a day. As your small changes become habit, you can continue to add more healthy choices. For example, choose just one of the following diet changes to start. Work on it for a few weeks, then add another and so on.

To set yourself up for success, try to keep things simple. Eating a healthier diet doesn't have to be complicated. Instead of being overly concerned with counting calories, for example, think of your diet in terms of color, variety, and freshness. Focus on avoiding packaged and processed foods and opting for more fresh ingredients whenever possible.

Prepare more of your own meals. Cooking more meals at home can help you take charge of what you're eating and better monitor exactly what goes into your food. You'll eat fewer calories and avoid the chemical additives, added sugar, and unhealthy fats of packaged and takeout foods that can leave you feeling tired, bloated, and irritable, and exacerbate symptoms of depression, stress, and anxiety.

Make the right changes. When cutting back on unhealthy foods in your diet, it's important to replace them with healthy alternatives. Replacing dangerous trans fats with healthy fats (such as switching fried chicken for grilled salmon) will make a positive difference to your health. Switching animal fats for refined carbohydrates, though (such as switching your breakfast bacon for a donut), won't lower your risk for heart disease or improve your mood.

Read the labels. It's important to be aware of what's in your food as manufacturers often hide large amounts of sugar or unhealthy fats in packaged food, even food claiming to be healthy.

Focus on how you feel after eating. This will help foster healthy new habits and tastes. The healthier the food you eat, the better you'll feel after a meal. The more junk food you eat, the more likely you are to feel uncomfortable, nauseous, or drained of energy.

Drink plenty of water. Water helps flush our systems of waste products and toxins, yet many of us go through life dehydrated—causing tiredness, low energy, and headaches.

It's common to mistake thirst for hunger, so staying well hydrated will also help you make healthier food choices.

It's not just what you eat, but when you eat.

Eat breakfast, and eat smaller meals throughout the day. A healthy breakfast can jumpstart your metabolism, while eating small, healthy meals keeps your energy up all day.

Avoid eating late at night. Try to eat dinner earlier and fast for 14-16 hours until breakfast the next morning. Studies suggest that eating only when you're most active and giving your digestive system a long break each day may help to regulate weight.

Add more fruit and vegetables to your diet. Fruit and vegetables are low in calories and nutrient dense, which means they are packed with vitamins, minerals, antioxidants, and fiber. Focus on eating the recommended daily amount of at least five servings of fruit and vegetables and it will naturally fill you up and help you cut back on unhealthy foods. A serving is half a cup of raw fruit or veg or a small apple or banana, for example. Most of us need to double the amount we currently eat.

Make your vegetables a mouth watering dish. Salads and steamed veggies can quickly become bland, there are plenty of ways to add taste to your vegetable dishes.

Add color. Not only do brighter, deeper colored vegetables contain higher concentrations of vitamins, minerals and antioxidants, but they can vary the flavor and make meals more visually appealing. Add color using fresh or sundried tomatoes, glazed carrots or beets, roasted red cabbage wedges, yellow squash, or sweet, colorful peppers.

Liven up salad greens. Branch out beyond lettuce. Kale, arugula, spinach, mustard greens, broccoli, and Chinese cabbage are all packed with nutrients. To add flavor to your salad greens, try drizzling with olive oil, adding a spicy dressing, or sprinkling with almond slices, chickpeas, a little bacon, parmesan, or goat cheese.

Satisfy your sweet tooth. Naturally sweet vegetables—such as carrots, beets, sweet potatoes, yams, onions, bell peppers, and squash—add sweetness to your meals and reduce your cravings for added sugar. Add them to soups, stews, or pasta sauces for a satisfying sweet kick.

Cook green beans, broccoli, Brussels sprouts, and asparagus in new ways. Instead of boiling or steaming these healthy sides, try grilling, roasting, or pan frying them with chili flakes, garlic, shallots, mushrooms, or onion. Or marinate in tangy lemon or lime before cooking.

Shop the perimeter of the grocery store

In general, healthy eating ingredients are found around the outer edges of most grocery stores, while the center aisles are filled with processed and packaged foods that aren't good for you. Shop the perimeter of the store for most of your groceries (fresh fruits and vegetables, fish and poultry, whole grain breads and dairy products), add a few things from the freezer section (frozen fruits and vegetables), and visit the aisles for spices, oils, and whole grains (like rolled oats, brown rice, whole wheat pasta).

Cook when you can. Try to cook one or both weekend days or on a weekday evening and make extra to freeze or set aside for another night. Cooking ahead saves time and money, and it is gratifying to know that you have a home cooked meal waiting to be eaten.

Challenge yourself to come up with two or three dinners that can be put together without going to the store—utilizing things in your pantry, freezer, and spice rack. A delicious dinner of whole grain pasta with a quick tomato sauce or a quick and easy black bean quesadilla on a whole wheat flour tortilla (among endless other recipes) could act as your go-to meal when you are just too busy to shop or cook.

Plan quick and easy meals ahead. Healthy eating starts with great planning. You will have won half the healthy diet battle if you have a well-stocked kitchen, a stash of quick and easy recipes, and plenty of healthy snacks.

Plan your meals by the week or even the month. One of the best ways to have a healthy diet is to prepare your own food and eat in regularly. Pick a few healthy recipes that you and your family like and build a meal schedule around them. If you have three or four meals planned per week and eat leftovers on the other nights, you will be much farther ahead than if you are eating out or having frozen dinners most nights.

Conclusion

Thank you again for downloading this book!

I hope this book was able to help you to learn one or two things on how to live a healthy lifestyle, what to eat, when to eat and so on.

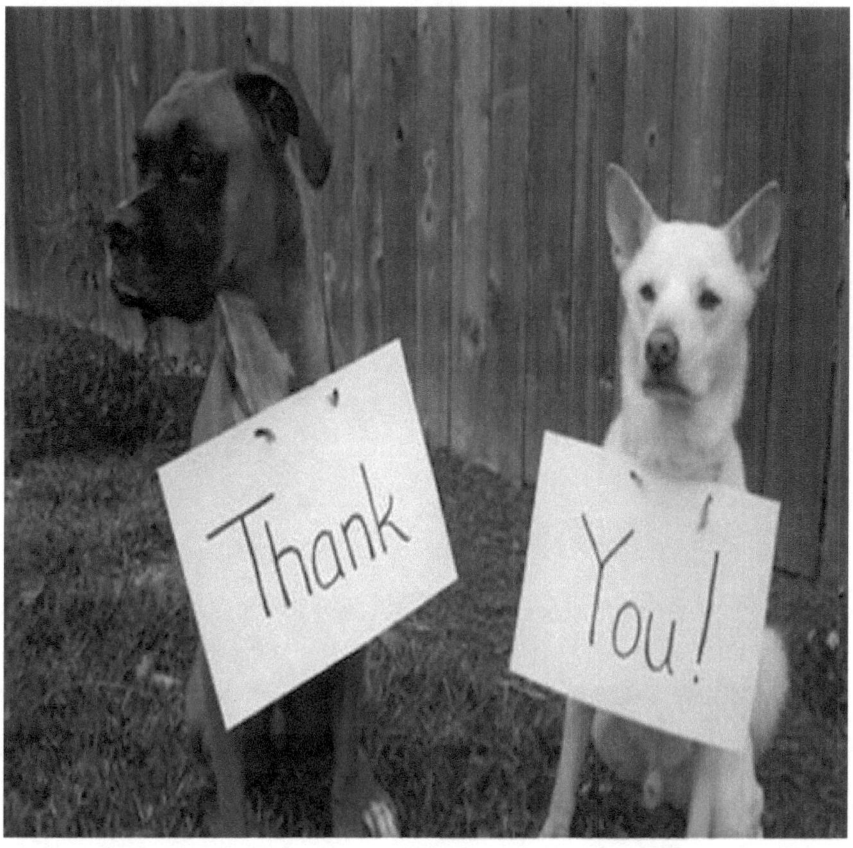

Finally, if you enjoyed this book, then I'd like to ask you for a favor, would you be kind enough to leave a review for this book on Amazon? It'd be greatly appreciated!

Thank you and good luck!